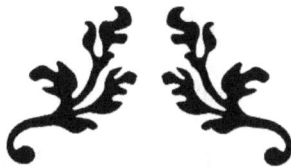

JUST A CLOSER WALK

90 Breath Prayers for the Healthcare Professional

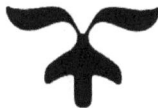

DIANA LEAGH MATTHEWS

Just a Closer Walk: Breath Prayers for the
Healthcare Professional
©2021 by Diana Leagh Matthews

ISBN-13: 978-1-7369727-1-7

Published by LynneLee Lane Publishing

Scripture quotations marked ESV are from The Holy
Bible, English Standard Version. ESV® Text
Edition: 2016. Copyright © 2001 by Crossway
Bibles, a publishing ministry of Good News
Publishers.

Copyedited by Bridget Halford

Dedicated to:

To all healthcare workers
You are essential

And to my Lord and Savior,
Jesus Christ for loving me and
guiding me~even when I
grumble about it.

Acknowledgements

This book would not be possible without the assistance and support of so many people.

From the beginning my Mastermind group-Arlene Mallet, Bridget Halfyard and Mary Harker—cheered my idea and continued encouraging me throughout the process until completion.

My WordGirls Summer Retreat group provided support and encouragement throughout the writing process. Gina Stinson and Lisa-Anne Wooldridge offered continued support and accountability throughout the remainder of the process.

Thank you to Bridget Halfyard for her editing expertise and overall heart and encouragement for the project.

Theresa Patten and Mary Lou Karas for your continued support, invaluable advice, and wisdom throughout the entire process. You let me bounce so many things off you and kept proofing and offering insight.

To Kathy Willis, my writing coach, for your continued guidance and answering my questions.

A big thank you to my prayer partners for their prayers over the years as we seek God in making publication possible.

Finally, to Cherry Grant, Dee Dee Parker and my mother, Sandy Allen. Thank you for your continuing wisdom, guidance and support through this journey and life in general.

To my father, Rev. Clarence Allen, who left us all too early. However, he instilled a love for senior adults, and those dealing with health issues into my heart from a young age.

And most importantly thank you to God Almighty, who has guided and directed me through this entire process. This project would not be possible without his help and wisdom.

Foreword

Working in healthcare, I have heard the daily stresses and frustrations various departments encounter.

This inspired the concept for this book. The prayers cover a wide range of issues and concerns various healthcare professionals face throughout their workday.

The prayers are purposely short for those on-the-go moments.

However, there is also room at the end of each prayer to journal, complete the action task or write your own prayer.

I pray these breath prayers will help you destress and draw closer to the Lord.

After all, the goal is to be the best we can be for our patients.

Blessings,

Leagh

P.S. Additional breath prayer books will soon be available for activity professionals, caregivers, and individuals dealing with healthcare issues.

TABLE OF CONTENTS

5   Prayers for Healthcare Professionals

7   Prayers for Healthcare Professionals

Prayer 1

PRAYER FOR A CONCERNED LOVED ONE

"Know this, my beloved brothers: let every person be quick to hear, slow to speak, slow to anger."
James 1:19

Lord, help me stop and listen. Sometimes all a loved one needs is someone to listen and hear what they are saying. Help me be the ear they need at this moment. Even when I am busy and the day quickly moves on, help me pause long enough to care. Sometimes all I need to do is be the person who shows I care by hearing the needs of others.

Action *Plan*:

Take five minutes and listen to
someone today.

Prayer 2

♡

PRAYER OVER AN UNCERTAIN FUTURE

"He made the storm be still, and the waves of the sea were hushed. Then they were glad that the waters were quiet, and he brought them to their desired haven."
Psalm 107:29-30

Lord, the future is uncertain, but we are promised that you are in control of our tomorrows. Calm my uncertainty and the fears about tomorrow to help me to take each day with one step at a time.

*A*ction *Plan*:

Take a deep breath and ask the
Lord to calm your fears and
nerves.

Prayer 3

PRAYER FOR A DIFFICULT PATIENT

"Do nothing from selfish ambition or conceit, but in humility count others more significant than yourselves. Let each of you look not only to his own interests, but also to the interests of others."
Philippians 2:3-4

Lord, give me the wisdom, guidance, and direction to deal with this person and their situation today. You know this individual's heart, as well as the crux of the matter. I pray you will provide me with the wisdom and guidance I need. Help me strive to do my best to meet thei.6r needs.

Action Plan:

Take five minutes to personally
connect with the patient. Talk
with them about a picture in
their room, a family member who
visited or the program on TV.

*P*rayer 4

PRAYER WHEN YOU NEED TO DELIVER DIFFICULT NEWS

"So also you have sorrow now, but I will see you again, and your hearts will rejoice, and no one will take your joy from you."

John 16:22

*L*ord, this is the part of my job I detest. Go before me, be with me and stay after me, as I gently deliver difficult news to my patient. Provide me with the words of comfort this person and their family need during this challenging time.

Action *Plan*:

Put yourself in the shoes of
your patient. What words and
actions would you need?

Prayer 5

PRAYER WHEN A PATIENT DOESN'T KNOW GOD

"And let us not grow weary of doing good, for in due season we will reap, if we do not give up."
Galatians 6:9

Lord, only you know the true condition of a person's heart. I see this person struggling with the events in their lives and battling spiritual matters. I pray you will work miracles in their life. We place our trust in you as only you know when the harvest is ready. Show me how to be an example of your love for this patient. May seeds be

planted and harvested in your
time and in your way.

Action *Plan*:

Ask God to reveal at least one
person to pray for this week.
Lift them up to Jesus as you go
throughout your day.

*P*rayer 6

PRAYER FOR DEALING WITH A DIFFICULT FAMILY MEMBER

"Above all, keep loving one another earnestly, since love covers a multitude of sins."
1 Peter 4:8

*L*ord, this family member is driving me crazy. You know their situation and their heart even when I do not. I lift this patient to you for healing and peace while I tend to their physical needs. Use my servant heart in a way that will reflect your mighty power and glory in their life, leading them closer to you.

*A*ction *Plan*:

Pray for this person
specifically by name as you go
throughout the day.

Prayer 7

PRAYER FOR A HURTING PATIENT

"He heals the brokenhearted and binds up their wounds."
Psalm 147:3

Lord, there are many patients struggling with physical, emotional, and mental pain. I lift them up to you as the Great Physician and healer to provide comfort and peace.

⚜

Action *Plan*:

Pray specifically for someone
you know is hurting. If
possible, visit, call, or text
them to ensure they feel cared
for.

Prayer 8

PRAYER WHEN SHORT STAFFED

*"And a second is like it: You shall love
your neighbor as yourself."*
Matthew 22:39

Lord, once again we are short staffed. My workload is already stretched beyond my comfort zone. My coworkers and I are doing the best we can, but our patients still suffer. Many patients and family members do not understand the load thrust upon us. Help me keep my eyes on you as I serve my patients with a heart of compassion. I cannot get through this shift without you.

✻

Action *Plan*:

Imagine you are serving God with
each patient.

Prayer 9

PRAYER FOR COMPLAINING CO-WORKERS

"Peace I leave with you; my peace I give to you. Not as the world gives do I give to you. Let not your hearts be troubled, neither let them be afraid."
John 14:27

Lord, all around me I hear grumbling and complaining from co-workers. There always seems to be something to criticize. Help me keep my eyes and heart on you as I tune out the negativity surrounding my workplace. I pray you will work in the heart and lives of all who enter my workplace. Teach me

to use my servant heart and
attitude to maintain peace with
everyone I interact with today.

Action *Plan*:

Compliment someone today.

Prayer 10

PRAYER FOR A DIFFICULT BOSS

"Do not be anxious about anything, but in everything by prayer and supplication with thanksgiving let your requests be made known to God."
Philippians 4:6

Lord, my boss is making my work life exceedingly difficult. There are too many demands, nitpicking, an overbearing spirit, and other issues that only you understand. Help me to consistently do my best. I pray for my boss and whatever is going on in their life. I lift them up to you and humbly ask for peace, guidance, and comfort.

Action *Plan*:

```
Pray for your boss each time you
interact with them regardless of
the added stress they put on
your job.
```

Prayer 11

PRAYER FOR DIFFICULT CO-WORKER

"God is our refuge and strength, a very present help in trouble."
Psalm 46:1

Lord, I am so frustrated I could scream. My co-workers are making my work situation difficult. I do not know what to do and I am not sure how much more I can take. Help me through this difficult time. Teach me to pray for my co-worker even when we are surrounded by conflict. You know what is going on in their life and heart. I lift them up to you and ask for a mighty work

to be done in their lives by
your Holy Spirit.

❀

Action *Plan*:

Make an extra effort to be kind
to the person and pray for them
as you want to be prayed for.

Prayer 12

PRAYER WHEN SACRIFICING TIME FOR WORK

"Whoever brings blessing will be enriched, and one who waters will himself be watered."
Proverbs 11:25

Lord, it is frustrating when I have to sacrifice my rest days to work. Yet, I care deeply for my patients. Help me to go about my day with a heart for you serving my patients with a joyful spirit. Give me guidance and direction in finding balance between home life and work life. Help me set healthy professional boundaries so that my personal life and health do not suffer.

❦

Action *Plan*:

```
Set healthy boundaries and write
them down. Refer to them when
you are asked to stretch your
limits.
```

Prayer 13

PRAYER WHEN WORKING A HOLIDAY

"Only fear the Lord and serve him faithfully with all your heart. For consider what great things he has done for you."
1 Samuel 12:24

Lord, a frustrating part of health care is sacrificing the holiday{s} and time with family to care for our patients. I would much rather be home with loved ones on this special day, instead of at work. Help me treat each patient with the respect and care my loved ones would receive from me. I am sure they also long to be home with their family. Help me love them as you love me and teach me to

spread joy in their lives on
this holiday.

Action *Plan*:

Do something special for both
yourself and your patients.

Prayer 14

PRAYER FOR A
PATIENT'S NEEDS

*"The Lord is near to the brokenhearted
and saves the crushed in spirit."
Psalm 34:18*

Lord, all around me I see need
and hurting hearts and bodies.
You know my patient's needs;
please reveal to me the best way
to care for each of them. I pray
they will see your unconditional
love. I ask you to strengthen
and heal their pain.

❀

Action *Plan*:

Spend a few minutes today
dedicated to a prayer walk on
your floor or area.

Prayer 15

PRAYER TO LOVE
PATIENT

*"A new commandment I give to you, that
you love one another: just as I have
loved you, you also are to love one
another."*
John 13:34

Lord, help me love my patients
like you do. Remind me to be an
example of your love to each
person I meet today. Thank you
for the ultimate sacrifice you
paid for each of us to live in
peace and love.

*A*ction *Plan*:

Listen to Casting Crowns song
"Love them like Jesus".

Prayer 16

PRAYER FOR HELPING
AN ALZHEIMER'S
PATIENT

"With all humility and gentleness, with patience, bearing with one another in love."
Ephesians 4:2

Lord, this disease called Alzheimer's is terrible. I do not know how much more I can stand. I have repeated myself over and over until I'm at my wits end. I know they are doing their best, but my stamina is depleting. Help me to be patient, and kind to this individual. I cannot imagine what they must be experiencing. Give me the strength and wisdom

to care for them with the
dignity and respect I would want
if our roles were reversed. Help
me treat them in the manner I
would want to be treated if the
roles were reversed.

❦

Action Plan:

Take a deep breath and imagine,
even for a minute, what it would
be like to be in the shoes of an
Alzheimer's patient.

Prayer 17

PRAYER WHEN WORKING ON FRONT LINES

"Rejoice in hope, be patient in tribulation, be constant in prayer."
Romans 12:12

Lord, we are on the front line helping many people in desperate need. The magnitude of patients who need our attention is overwhelming. Give our team the strength to keep going when we are depleted of energy. Help us provide the best care possible even when it feels we have nothing left to give.

Action *Plan*:

Take five minutes for yourself
and take in a deep breath of
fresh air.

Prayer 18

PRAYER DURING A PANDEMIC

"Behold, I am with you and will keep you wherever you go, and will bring you back to this land. For I will not leave you until I have done what I have promised you."
Genesis 28:15

Lord, as we work through this overwhelming worldwide pandemic, we ask for safety and serenity as we attend to the daily needs of our patients. Diminish our personal fear so we can walk with the strength and wisdom needed to provide the best care for our patients.

Action Plan:

Stand somewhere quiet and fill
your lungs with three slow,
deep, healing breaths.

Prayer 19

PRAYER WHEN EXHAUSTED

"Come to me, all who labor and are heavy laden, and I will give you rest."
Matthew 11:28

Lord, we have been working long hours and I am exhausted. You promise when we are weary you will provide strength. I am leaning into you and your strength to make it through the remainder of my shift.

Action Plan:

Sing or listen to "Leaning on the Everlasting Arms".

Prayer 20

PRAYER WHEN FACING FEARS

"Keep your life free from love of money, and be content with what you have, for he has said, "I will never leave you nor forsake you." So we can confidently say, "The Lord is my helper; I will not fear; what can man do to me?"
Hebrews 13:5-6

Lord, we are working through a crisis that is beyond anything we have experienced in the past. The circumstances attract many co-workers to depend on my leadership, but I am battling my own fear. Remind me to put my trust in you when I am afraid.

Action *Plan*:

When your fear sneaks in repeat
the phrase: "The Lord is my
helper, I will not be afraid."

Prayer 21

PRAYER DURING A CRISIS

"Do not be anxious about anything, but in everything by prayer and supplication with thanksgiving let your requests be made known to God."
Philippians 4:6

Lord, we are in a crisis. It is scary and exhausting. Give me the guidance, wisdom, and direction to provide the best possible care for our patients. Walk with us through this time and help us remember we are never alone.

Action *Plan*:

```
Take a deep breath and count
backwards from ten.
```

Prayer 22

PRAYER TO SEE THE PERSON INSTEAD OF THE ILLNESS

"But the Lord said to Samuel, "Do not look on his appearance or on the height of his stature, because I have rejected him. For the Lord sees not as man sees: man looks on the outward appearance, but the Lord looks on the heart." 1 Samuel 16:7

Lord, help me see the person before me and not the illness. It is so easy to desensitize myself in this profession. You have placed human lives in my hand. They are afraid and have questions about their uncertain future. Help me provide the

guidance and assurance they
need. Prepare my words with the
compassion that I would need in
this situation.

Action *Plan*:

What is the one thing you would
need to hear in this situation
if the roles were reversed?

Prayer 23

PRAYER IN A CRISIS

"Therefore do not be anxious about tomorrow, for tomorrow will be anxious for itself. Sufficient for the day is its own trouble."
Matthew 6:34

Lord, due to unforeseen circumstances our space cannot accommodate the over flux of patients and their needs. We have resorted to using makeshift cots and our resources for care are being stretched thin. We ask you to help us keep our eyes, minds and hearts on our patients and their needs.

Action *Plan*:

When things become stressful,
remind yourself you are working
for Jesus.

Prayer 24

PRAYER WHEN
DESPERATELY NEEDING
GOD

*"The God who equipped me with
strength and made my way blameless."*
Psalm 18:32

Lord, we ask for guidance,
wisdom, and direction during
this difficult and challenging
time.

☙❧

Action *Plan*:

Lean into God and seek Him.

*P*rayer 25

♡

PRAYER TO OVERCOME FEAR

*"Casting all your anxieties on him,
because he cares for you."*
1 Peter 5:7

*L*ord, Florence Nightingale said, "little can be done under the spirit of fear". You know my current fear, and I cast it upon you. I humbly ask that you take my fear and give me the strength to move forward as I care for others who are hurting physically and spiritually.

Action *Plan*:

Take a deep breath and then take
the first step.

Prayer 26

PRAYER WHEN WE DON'T FEEL WE CAN GO ON

"Come to me, all who labor and are heavy laden, and I will give you rest."
Matthew 11:28

Lord, we are exhausted and weary, physically, mentally, and emotionally. Give us the strength to carry on and provide the best care possible to our patients.

✾

*A*ction *Plan*:

Take a few minutes {whether 5
minutes, an hour, or a day} for
yourself and schedule a vacation
as soon as possible. Take a deep
breath and relax.

Prayer 27

PRAYER TO TREAT OTHERS WITH COMPASSION

"And as you wish that others would do to you, do so to them."
Luke 6:31

Lord, help me remember to treat each person with the compassion and understanding I would expect to receive. I may not understand what they are going through, but I can reflect your love through my actions.

Action *Plan*:

Pray for someone who challenges
your personal patience.

Prayer 28

PRAYER TO MAKE PATIENT COMFORTABLE

"Do not neglect the gift you have…"
1 Timothy 4:14

Lord, show me ways to make the patient more comfortable. Reveal to me ways I can make patients feel at home in their room. May I have the foresight to know how to comfort this patient physically and emotionally.

Action Plan:

Think about how you would like
to be treated if you were this
patient.

Prayer 29

PRAYER FOR PATIENTS

"And this is the confidence that we have toward him, that if we ask anything according to his will he hears us."
1 John 5:14

Lord, help me lift to you in prayer each patient in my care. Even if it is silently as they walk through the door or while I am going about my duties and providing care. Give me a spirit of prayer.

Action Plan:

Designate a time to silently pray for everything you do during that period.

Prayer 30

PRAYER FOR A HEARTBROKEN FAMILY

*"He heals the brokenhearted and binds
up their wounds."*
Psalm 147:3

Lord, part of my job is dealing with heartbroken families. While this is only a patient to me, it is someone's parent, child, sibling, spouse, friend or loved one. Give me the wisdom and words to provide comfort to the family. Help me know when the best communication is a hug, a gentle hand on the arm or to just be present with them during this difficult and trying time.

Action *Plan*:

Take time to listen.

Prayer 31

PRAYER FOR CLEAR
COMMUNICATION

*"Know this, my beloved brothers: let
every person be quick to hear, slow to
speak, slow to anger."*
James 1:19

*L*ord, help me have clear
communication with the patient
and their family. Sadly,
patients often feel they are not
properly informed. Help me be
honest and transparent when
sharing information with
patients about their care.

Action *Plan*:

Have a heart and ears to listen.
Count to ten before speaking.

Prayer 32

PRAYER WHEN I DON'T FEEL I HAVE ENOUGH TO GIVE

"And we know that for those who love God all things work together for good, for those who are called according to his purpose."
Romans 8:28

Lord, I give my best to my patients, but there are days when I wonder what I have accomplished. I often feel I am not making a difference in their lives or I am not doing enough. I know my personal limits and that I can only do so much. Please intervene to show me those who truly need my

assistance and help me make a
difference in their lives.

☙

Action *Plan*:

Ask the Lord to show you how you
are making a difference and/or
to send you to someone who needs
you.

Prayer 33

PRAYER OF THANKS

"For God is not unjust so as to overlook your work and the love that you have shown for his name in serving the saints, as you still do."
Hebrews 6:10

Lord, thank you for the opportunity to serve others through this difficult time in their lives. Give me the strength to continue serving you with all my skills and talents.

Action *Plan*:

Reflect on your day and look for
signs of God's presence.

Prayer 34

PRAYER TO OVERCOME
DISCOURAGEMENT

"So we do not lose heart..."
2 Corinthians 4:16

Lord, I am discouraged by staff
who are not supportive of our
daily service to our patients.
Remove my negativity and the
discouraged attitude sparked by
others. Change my heart in
dealing with staff who are less
than supportive of what we do.
Help me to show your love to
others. I cannot change their
actions but can change mine.

Action *Plan*:

Pray for a staff member who
bothers you.

Prayer 35

PRAYER WHEN DEALING WITH A DIFFICULT FAMILY

"Be strong and courageous. Do not fear or be in dread of them, for it is the Lord your God who goes with you. He will not leave you or forsake you."
Deuteronomy 31:6

Lord, there is a difficult family and/or family dynamic in our midst we are having to deal with. As I face this challenge, help me guard my mouth and provide discernment when dealing with each person involved. May you be given the glory in all I do and say as this situation comes to a resolution.

Action *Plan*:

Take a deep breath, say a quick
prayer and the initiative to
approach a difficult person.

Prayer 36

PRAYER TO DEAL WITH STRESS

"Casting all your anxieties on him, because he cares for you."
1 Peter 5:7

Lord, I am stressed. There is a lot of responsibility on my shoulders, and it is taking a toll on my physical and mental health. You know the issues. Help me to keep my eyes on you as I search for the wisdom, guidance, and direction through this difficult time. Your shoulders are so much bigger than mine and I cast this burden on you.

✤

Action *Plan*:

Imagine casting your burdens on
the Lord and when possible take
a few hours to go fishing or do
something relaxing and peaceful.

Prayer 37

PRAYER WHEN EXHAUSTED

"The Lord is my strength and my song, and he has become my salvation; this is my God, and I will praise him, my father's God, and I will exalt him."
Exodus 15:2

Lord, I am so exhausted I cannot see straight. The days have been long and tedious. I need time to rest now but our schedule does not allow for the break. Give me the strength I need to keep going. It is not by my own power but in your mighty power that I am able to push through.

Action Plan:

Take ten deep breaths and if possible, go outside for five minutes of fresh air.

Prayer 38

PRAYER WHEN OVERWHELMED

*"But Jesus looked at them and said,
"With man this is impossible, but with
God all things are possible."*
Matthew 19:26

Lord, I am overwhelmed with the situation at hand. I have never seen anything like this. I humbly ask for the guidance and wisdom only you can provide. Lead me to the answers I need during this time and in this situation.

*A*ction *Plan*:

Ask the Lord to guide you to the
answer or send someone alongside
to assist.

Prayer 39

PRAYER OVER THE LOSS OF A PATIENT

"He will wipe away every tear from their eyes, and death shall be no more, neither shall there be mourning, nor crying, nor pain anymore, for the former things have passed away."
Revelation 21:4

Lord, it is so difficult to lose a patient. Whether it is someone we just met or someone we had a longstanding relationship with. The sting and pain still exist as we grieve this loss. You know this individual and their heart, as well as those loved ones who survive. Into your hands we commit their spirit and lift our

prayers for comfort and strength
to all those left behind.

✿

Action *Plan*:

What is one lesson you learned
from this person or this loss?

Prayer 40

PRAYER FOR SENSITIVITY TO OTHERS

"With all humility and gentleness, with patience, bearing with one another in love."
Ephesians 4:2

Lord, there are days I want to scream in frustration because someone is so demanding. However, I have no idea what they may be going through. I pray for your comfort and peace to come over this person. Help me be sensitive to their needs and remind me that I am serving you. May others see you in me as I interact with this patient.

Action *Plan*:

```
Pray for this person every time
you walk in the room.
```

Prayer 41

PRAYER FOR A DIFFICULT DECISION

"In all your ways acknowledge him, and he will make straight your paths."
Proverbs 3:6

Lord, I have a big decision to make. You know the path you have for me and everyone else involved in this situation. Give me wisdom and guidance to make a good decision. As I keep my eyes on you. I ask for you to provide overwhelming peace about this decision.

Action *Plan*:

Make a list of pros and cons and
if possible, talk the situation
over with a valued mentor.

Prayer 42

PRAYER FOR UNCERTAIN TIMES

"But Jesus looked at them and said,
"With man this is impossible, but with
God all things are possible."
Matthew 19:26

Lord, I am at a loss about what to do. This is beyond my capability, but I know all things are possible with you. Send the help and assistance I need to make the most informed decision possible. Open my eyes and heart to the answer.

❦ Action *Plan*:

Ask a colleague or specialists
for their insight and opinion.

Prayer 43

PRAYER WHEN
DELIVERING BAD NEWS

*"Now may our Lord Jesus Christ himself,
and God our Father, who loved us and
gave us eternal comfort and good hope
through grace, comfort your hearts and
establish them in every good work and
word."*
2 Thessalonians 2:16-17

Lord, the worst part of my job
is having to give bad news. I
lift this person to you, even
before I speak to them. Give
them the comfort and strength
needed for the plans you have
for them. Give me the wisdom and
guidance needed to share this
news and if necessary, implement
the next steps toward their

care. Into your hands I commit their care.

Action Plan:

Imagine how you would want to hear this news if it were about your health. Be compassionate.

Prayer 44

PRAY WHEN FEELING OVERWHELMED AND STRETCHED

"He gives power to the faint, and to him who has no might he increases strength."
Isaiah 40:29

Lord, I am frazzled, weary and stretched too thin. I do not know how much longer I can go on at this pace. Strengthen and restore me as I find a way out of this desert land.

*A*ction *Plan*:

Make it a habit to take a daily
walk.

Prayer 45

PRAYER TO BE A LIGHT IN THE WORLD

"In the same way, let your light shine before others, so that they may see your good works and give glory to your Father who is in heaven."
Matthew 5:16

Lord, help me stay upbeat during this difficult and trying time. Help me keep my eyes set on you so others will see a reflection of you within me. Allow me to be a light in this dark world so I may motivate and inspire those around me.

Action *Plan*:

Each day recite five things you are thankful for.

Prayer 46

PRAYER TO BE AN INSTRUMENT OF PEACE

"Have I not commanded you? Be strong and courageous. Do not be frightened, and do not be dismayed, for the Lord your God is with you wherever you go."
Joshua 1:9

Lord, make me an instrument of your peace. Show me how to love others as you love them. Teach me to serve others with a heart set on you.

*A*ction *Plan*:

Ask the Lord to show you who to
serve and show His love today.

*P*rayer 47

PRAYER FOR A HURTING SOUL

"Ask, and it will be given to you; seek, and you will find; knock, and it will be opened to you."
Matthew 7:7

*L*ord, I lift this individual to you. The world around them is hurting not only physically, but also mentally and emotionally. You know all the hurt and pain, regardless of the type or size. Work in their life and show your love as only you can. Plant the seeds so this person will have no doubt you love them and have not forsaken them.

*A*ction *Plan*:

Offer to pray with them or read
scripture to them.

Prayer 48

PRAYER FOR THE LOST

"For God so loved the world, that he gave his only Son, that whoever believes in him should not perish but have eternal life."
John 3:16

Lord, I pray for this individual who is lost. You know the seeds which have been planted and when the harvest is ripe. Help me to be both a seed planter and harvester, as you deem fit. Burden their heart to draw closer to you so they may come to know and love you.

Action *Plan*:

Pray for this individual to come
to know Christ.

Prayer 49

PRAYER WHEN A
PATIENT ISN'T HONEST

*"For nothing is hidden that will not be
made manifest, nor is anything secret
that will not be known and come to
light."*
Luke 8:17

Lord, there is a patient who is
not being honest about their
needs. This makes it difficult
for our staff to know how to
help them. Give us guidance and
direction to know how to best
care for this person. Help us to
know how best to serve the needs
of this individual despite what
is being hidden from us.

❀

*A*ction *Plan*:

Take a moment to have a friendly
conversation with the patient.

Prayer 50

PRAYER WHEN A MISTAKE IS MADE

"Better is a poor man who walks in his integrity than a rich man who is crooked in his ways."
Proverbs 28:6

Lord, I have made a huge mistake in my duties. It is not on purpose, but it was a costly mistake. Give me the guidance, wisdom, and direction to know how to best handle this situation. Help me speak truth and walk in integrity regardless of the outcome. I give you all the honor and glory.

Action *Plan*:

Speak with honesty and walk with
integrity.

Prayer 51

PRAYER WHEN A
PATIENT IS IN DANGER

*"But understand this, that in the last days
there will come times of difficulty...But as
for you, continue in what you have
learned and have firmly believed,
knowing from whom you learned it."*
2 Timothy 3:1, 14

Lord, my patient is in danger or
in a harmful situation. Give me
a heart of compassion and wisdom
to know how best to approach
this situation. I lift my
patient to you and ask you to
help them be honest with me.
Give me guidance to know how
best to handle this issue and
whether additional resources
should be called upon.

Action *Plan*:

Listen to the patient and watch
their body language.

Prayer 52

PRAYER WHEN DEALING WITH BUREAUCRACY

"They have deeply corrupted themselves as in the days of Gibeah: he will remember their iniquity; he will punish their sins."
Hosea 9:9

Lord, there are times when the entire system seems broken and full of bureaucratic nonsense. Help me keep my eyes and heart on my mission to put my patients first in all things. As I traverse this system remind me of my passion for the medical field and guide and direct me to

focus on you as the Great
Physician.

✻

Action *Plan*:

Research and discover if there
are work-a-rounds or another
answer.

Prayer 53

PRAYER OVER AN OPPRESSIVE SPIRIT

"Whoever oppresses the poor to increase his own wealth, or gives to the rich, will only come to poverty."
Proverbs 22:16-17

Lord, there is an oppressive spirit in this place. I do not know how this is happening, but I ask for your light and truth to shine through. Strengthen me to stand against opposition as an example of your love. In all things, I give you all the praise and glory.

Action *Plan*:

Walk the halls and pray for the
people in patient rooms and/or
offices.

Prayer 54

PRAYER TO PROVIDE THE BEST POSSIBLE CARE

"In all things I have shown you that by working hard in this way we must help the weak and remember the words of the Lord Jesus, how he himself said, 'It is more blessed to give than to receive.'"
Acts 20:35

Lord, help me remember the Hippocratic oath I took as I serve my patients to the best of my ability. Give me wisdom and guidance as I provide the best treatment possible to all my patients. Above all, help me keep my eyes on you.

Action *Plan*:

Repeat the Hippocratic Oath.

Prayer 55

PRAYER TO BE A GOOD LEADER

"Remember your leaders, those who spoke to you the word of God. Consider the outcome of their way of life, and imitate their faith."
Hebrews 13:7

Lord, being a leader is not always easy, whether in an unofficial or official capacity. Help me to lead with honor and integrity as I attempt to set a Godly example for everyone I meet.

Action *Plan*:

Make a list of your strengths.
How can you become a better
leader?

Prayer 56

PRAYER DURING A CRISIS

"Then they cried to the Lord in their trouble, and he delivered them from their distress. He made the storm be still, and the waves of the sea were hushed. Then they were glad that the waters were quiet, and he brought them to their desired haven."
Psalm 107:28-30

Lord, we are in the middle of a crisis. You know this crisis and the intricacies of the issues involved. We pray for guidance and wisdom in this situation. Guide and direct our steps and show us how to walk with integrity.

Action *Plan*:

Discuss the issue with mentors
or advisors.

Prayer 57

PRAYER FOR A SERVANT'S HEART

"For even the Son of Man came not to be served but to serve, and to give his life as a ransom for many."
Mark 10:45

Lord, give me a servant's heart as I care for my patients. Help me be the embodiment of you and provide the best care possible.

*A*ction *Plan*:

Imagine you are serving Jesus as you serve each patient.

Prayer 58

PRAYER WHEN TIME TO MOVE ON

*"Be strong and courageous. Do not fear
or be in dread of them, for it is the Lord
your God who goes with you. He will not
leave you or forsake you."*
Deuteronomy 31:6

Lord, the time has come for me
to leave my patients. They have
become so special to me and are
like family. I'm going to miss
them terribly, but at the same
time I'm excited for the new
adventure ahead. While I am
leaving, you will never leave
nor forsake them. I pray you
will send someone who loves and
cherishes them more than I do
and that in the days ahead you

will be with them and watch over
them in all things.

✸

Action *Plan*:

Take a Prayer Walk for patients.

Prayer 59

PRAYER OVER
CHANGES

"The Lord is my light and my salvation;
whom shall I fear? The Lord is the
stronghold of my life; of whom shall I be
afraid?"
Psalm 27:1

Lord, there are changes happening in our workplace from the top Administrators. Right now, there is a lot of uncertainty and fear. Help us trust you as only you know what the future holds. You know these changes and how they will affect all of us. Give us guidance, wisdom, and direction to best know how to move forward.

Action *Plan*:

Make a list of pros and cons.
What can you live with and what
becomes a game changer for you?

Prayer 60

PRAYER FOR TEAMWORK

"If the whole body were an eye, where would be the sense of hearing? If the whole body were an ear, where would be the sense of smell? But as it is, God arranged the members in the body, each one of them, as he chose. If all were a single member, where would the body be? As it is, there are many parts, yet one body."
1 Corinthians 12:17-20

Lord, this field of work requires teamwork. Both on our immediate team and our larger team. Help us as we learn to work together and compliment one another's strengths.

Action *Plan*:

How can you complement one
another? Read the book *The 5
Languages of Appreciation in the
Workplace.*

Prayer 61

PRAYER TO TAKE ONE DAY AT A TIME

"I can do all things through him who
strengthens me."
Philippians 4:13

Lord, help me to take one day at a time. No matter how crazy things become or how frustrated life gets. When I want to throw in the towel help me keep my eyes on you. There are times when it feels impossible to carry on, but then something happens to place a smile on my heart and remind me of the rewards. While I cannot do this alone, I know that I can do all things through you, because you

give me strength. Give me
strength now.

Action *Plan*:

Take a deep breath and go for a
long walk.

Prayer 62

PRAYER TO PROVIDE MOTIVATION

"Fear not, for I am with you; be not dismayed, for I am your God; I will strengthen you, I will help you, I will uphold you with my righteous right hand."
Isaiah 41:10

Lord, our staff and patients need to be motivated and rejuvenated. Give me guidance and wisdom to know how to spread joy, lift spirits and motivate them during this time. You know what each person needs, even when I do not. I place the situation into your hands and ask you to use me as an instrument of your love, peace, and joy.

Action Plan:

Read Galatians 5 and meditate on the fruits of the spirit. Determine how to implement this teaching into your workplace and/or own life.

Prayer 63

PRAYER TO EMPATHIZE WITH A PATIENT

"In the same way, let your light shine before others, so that they may see your good works and give glory to your Father who is in heaven."
Matthew 5:16

Lord, help me to put myself in my patient's shoes. Give me the heart and empathy to understand whatever they may be dealing with at this point. Help me shine your light into their lives.

Action *Plan*:

```
Close your eyes and imagine how
you would feel in their place
for a moment.
```

Prayer 64

PRAYER WHEN A PATIENT IS STRUGGLING

"So whatever you wish that others would do to you, do also to them, for this is the Law and the Prophets."
Matthew 7:12

Lord, this patient is having a difficult time. I do not understand what they are dealing with, but you know the struggle. Remind me to treat this person the way I would want to be treated. Whatever is going on in their life is no secret to you. Wrap your loving arms around this person and help them feel your comfort and embrace.

Action *Plan*:

Treat the patient the way you
would want to be treated. Even
if your kindness goes
unappreciated.

Prayer 65

PRAYER IN A LIFE AND DEATH SITUATION

"Be strong and courageous. Do not fear or be in dread of them, for it is the Lord your God who goes with you. He will not leave you or forsake you."
Deuteronomy 31:6

Lord, I am facing a challenging life and death situation. Guide and direct my steps, actions, and words. You know the situation and I ask you to go before me, walk beside me through this and stay after my physical job is complete. You know the fears and uncertainty being faced and promise to never leave nor forsake us.

*A*ction *Plan*:

Repeat "When I am afraid, I will
put my trust you in".

Prayer 66

PRAYER WHEN A PATIENT IS AFRAID

"Then they cried to the Lord in their trouble, and he delivered them from their distress."
Psalm 107: 6

Lord, I see fear in my patient's eyes, and it is heartbreaking. I lift this child of yours up to you. Be with them and provide them comfort like only you can. Show me little ways that I can help ease the burden on this precious child of yours.

Action *Plan*:

Find one special thing to do for
this individual.

Prayer 67

PRAYER WHEN A PATIENT IS DYING

"My flesh and my heart may fail, but God is the strength of my heart and my portion forever."
Psalm 73:26

Lord, it is difficult sitting here watching this precious individual as their life slowly ebbs from them. I lift this person up to you and ask you to provide comfort and peace in their final breaths. Help make their transition as peaceful and smooth as possible. May they feel your love and your presence beside them.

Action *Plan*:

Turn on some music to softly
play in the background.

Prayer 68

♡

PRAYER WHEN A DOOR CLOSES ON CAREER

"For I know the plans I have for you, declares the Lord, plans for welfare and not for evil, to give you a future and a hope."
Jeremiah 29:11

Lord, one door has closed in my career. Whether planned or unplanned it is difficult to say goodbye. I trust the plans you have for me will be filled with the guidance, direction, and wisdom I need moving forward. Open the doors for me and show me how to walk in your will for my life.

Action *Plan*:

Take a day to rest and seek the
Lord's direction for your life.

Prayer 69

PRAYER WHEN I DON'T FEEL LIKE A SUPERHERO

"Do not be conformed to this world, but be transformed by the renewal of your mind, that by testing you may discern what is the will of God, what is good and acceptable and perfect."
Romans 12:2

Lord, I do not feel like the superhero the rest of the world says I am. Help me see myself the way you see me. My goal is to keep my eyes on you as I do the best for my patients in all I do.

❦

*A*ction *Plan*:

List all the ways in which you
make a difference.

Prayer 70

PRAYER OF THANKSGIVING FOR TEAM

"Be kind to one another, tenderhearted, forgiving one another, as God in Christ forgave you."
Ephesians 4:32

Lord, I am extremely proud of our team. Thank you for the opportunity to work with this wonderful group of people. Help us continue to work together as we serve others. Help me express my appreciation to this group and show them how special they are to me.

❀

*A*ction *Plan*:

What is one special thing you
can do for your team?

Prayer 71

PRAYER WHEN DELIVERING DIFFICULT NEWS

"I lift up my eyes to the hills. From where does my help come? My help comes from the Lord, who made heaven and earth."
Psalm 121:1-2

Lord, it is time to give a patient and his/her family some difficult news. Guide and direct my words during this challenging time. Wrap your arms around them and help them feel your comfort and love. We do not understand why this is happening; I ask that you assist this family with

knowing the promise you give to
never leave nor forsake us.

❋

Action *Plan*:

Recite Psalm 23 to yourself as
you approach the family.

Prayer 72

PRAYER WHEN
FEELING OVERLOOKED

*"The eyes of the Lord are in every place,
keeping watch on the evil and the good."*
Proverbs 15:3

Lord, there are times when we feel our supervisors or administrators overlook or ignore the contribution our team or colleagues make. It is so difficult when we feel as if we do not matter. However, we are the ones who provide hands on care. Help us to hold our head high and keep our eyes on you. Even when others do not see all that we do, you see it and you know our hearts. Thank you for seeing and knowing all.

Action *Plan*:

Find a way to celebrate yourself
and the difference you make.

Prayer 73

PRAYER TO PROVIDE QUALITY CARE

"Then he said to his disciples, "The harvest is plentiful, but the laborers are few; therefore pray earnestly to the Lord of the harvest to send out laborers into his harvest."
Matthew 9:37-38

Lord, help me provide the best quality of care for my patients. When I am tired or weak, I lean on you for strength and energy. Show me how to exude your love and joy for these precious souls entrusted to me.

Action *Plan*:

Treat each patient with the same
respect, dignity, and attention
that you would for your own
loved one.

Prayer 74

PRAYER WHEN LOSE SOMEONE CLOSE

"He heals the brokenhearted and binds up their wounds."
Psalm 147:3

Lord, it is so difficult when we lose someone close to us. You know how much we loved this person and how much we will miss them. We trust they are in a better place and ask for your comfort and provision. Cover our hearts as we deal with this loss and mourn for this precious soul. Thank you for the opportunity to have this precious individual in my life. We will never forget all they meant to us.

Action Plan:

Create a small memorial or hold
a special gathering to remember
the person you have lost.

Prayer 75

PRAYER WHEN
OVERWHELMINGLY
BUSY

*"Even to your old age I am he, and to
gray hairs I will carry you. I have made,
and I will bear; I will carry and will
save."*
Isaiah 46:4

Lord, there are days when I am
overwhelmingly busy. It feels
there are times when it never
stops, and I do not get a break.
Help me do all that needs to be
done and have the strength,
energy, and stamina to sustain
this pace. Remind me to take
care of myself and find a
healthy balance of work tasks.

Action *Plan*:

Think of a way to reward
yourself at the end of the day
and/or week.

Prayer 76

PRAYER WHEN
DEALING WITH A
FAMILY CRISIS

*"Casting all your anxieties on him,
because he cares for you."*
1 Peter 5:7

Lord, I am distracted with a
family crisis at home. Help me
to focus only on the task at
hand as I serve my patients here
at work. It is challenging for
me not to worry about my family.
You know what is going on and
the struggles and pain and I
need to give it all to you. Help
me focus on my patients
providing the best care
possible. While I care for them,

I will trust you to care for my family at home.

Action Plan:

Write a letter to God expressing your feeling of worry for your family and your patients.

Prayer 77

PRAYER WHEN BURNED OUT

"I am feeble and crushed; I groan because of the tumult of my heart."
Psalm 38:8

Lord, I am tired and burned out. Help me remember the reason I got into this field and the ways I make a difference. Show me how to recharge myself as I take care of my own needs while attending to the needs of my patients.

Action *Plan*:

Get away for a few days to
refresh and recharge your body
and soul. Find a peaceful place
to enjoy a favorite activity.

Prayer 78

PRAYER TO NAVIGATE HEALTHCARE SYSTEM

*"Who provides for the raven its prey,
when its young ones cry to God for help,
and wander about for lack of food?"*
Job 38:41

Lord, sometimes the changes in health care are frustrating. Particularly when we see a patient in need and their insurance will not cover the necessary care. You know the needs of this patient; I pray you will be with them and provide them with care for all their needs.

Action *Plan*:

Seek the advice of a
knowledgeable colleague who can
help navigate your patient
through the health care system.

Prayer 79

PRAYER WHEN I HAVE
A CONNECTION WITH
A PATIENT

*"Let what you say be simply 'Yes' or
'No'; anything more than this comes
from evil."*
Matthew 5:37

Lord, there are some patients
who capture my heart and I feel
such a connection with them.
Help me find a healthy balance
between caregiver and friend.
Lead me in professional, but
deeply caring relationships with
others.

Action Plan:

List your professional
boundaries and review them at
the start of each day. If you
feel as though you might be
crossing the line, remind
yourself of your own personal
code of ethics.

Prayer 80

PRAYER WHEN FACING RETIREMENT

"A good man leaves an inheritance to his children's children, but the sinner's wealth is laid up for the righteous."
Proverbs 13:22

Lord, the time has come to retire. It is bittersweet, but I am thankful for the opportunity to serve others for so long. Guide and direct my steps as I move into retirement. Lead me towards your will for my life as I step out of my career and into a change in pace. I look to you, Lord, for guidance and direction.

Action *Plan*:

```
Make a list of all the things
you would like to do when you
retire.
```

Prayer 81

PRAYER WHEN HEART BREAKS FOR A PATIENT

"Be kind to one another, tenderhearted, forgiving one another, as God in Christ forgave you."
Ephesians 4:32

Lord, there are times when I am overcome with emotion as I watch a patient struggle towards a better quality of life. My heart breaks for them and I cry as I feel for them in their pain. Allow me to lift this person up to you. Help me serve this person with emotional strength that can only come from you.

*A*ction *Plan*:

Take time to cry and to calm
your personal emotions. Spend
some extra time making your
patient feel special.

Prayer 82

♡

PRAYER WHEN FINANCES IMPACTS QUALITY OF CARE

"Consider the ravens: they neither sow nor reap, they have neither storehouse nor barn, and yet God feeds them. Of how much more value are you than the birds!"
Luke 12:24

Lord, sometimes it all boils down to money. It is so frustrating when quality care is interrupted because a patient cannot afford to pay, or their insurance won't cover the appropriate care needed. My heart breaks when this happens. I wish there were a way to help

these patients when they
struggle. Some of the stories
are so sad and heartbreaking.
Guide me towards any options I
may have to help those in need.

Action *Plan*:

Be willing to listen to the
patient and allow them to share.

Prayer 83

PRAYER WHEN I STRUGGLE WITH OWN HEALTH ISSUES

"I can do all things through him who strengthens me."
Philippians 4:13

Lord, while caring for others I am dealing with my own health issues. There are times when I must push through my own pain and issues while carrying out my work duties. Help me take care of myself and know my limits while I do my best for my patients. I stand on your promises that I can do all things through you because you give me strength.

*A*ction *Plan*:

```
Take more time to rest and talk
with your doctor about lifestyle
changes.
```

Prayer 84

PRAYER WHEN PATIENT CAN'T AFFORD MEDICAL CARE

"Why, even the hairs of your head are all numbered. Fear not; you are of more value than many sparrows."
Luke 12:7

Lord, my heart hurts for this patient who needs medical care they cannot pay for. It is heartbreaking. This person is hurting and without this procedure they could die. Give me the guidance and wisdom to know how to best help this person.

Action *Plan*:

Encourage patient to investigate
fund raising opportunities.

Prayer 85

PRAYER WHEN
OVERLOOKED BY
ADMINISTRATION

*"Cast your burden on the Lord, and he
will sustain you; he will never permit the
righteous to be moved."*
Psalm 55:22

Lord, we are lacking
administrative support. You know
all the issues and stress those
leading our organization must
face; it continues to feel we
are overlooked and ignored. We
lift it all to you and ask for
your will to be done.

*A*ction *Plan*:

Pray individually for the people
who work in administration.

Prayer 86

PRAYER FOR
SELF-CARE

"But they who wait for the Lord shall renew their strength; they shall mount up with wings like eagles; they shall run and not be weary; they shall walk and not faint."
Isaiah 40:31

Lord, to care for my patients, I must refresh myself. Help me find ways to provide self-care so I can be at my best while serving my patients. Reveal to me the areas where I need more balance in my life.

Action *Plan*:

```
Make a list of things you enjoy
doing and that recharge you.
Include a few new things you
would like to experience.
```

Prayer 87

PRAYER OVER BUDGET
CUTS

*"The young lions suffer want and
hunger; but those who seek the Lord lack
no good thing."*
Psalm 34:10

Lord, it is frustrating when
budget cuts interfere with the
care and/or services our
patients receive. Our patients
have such faith in us, but these
cuts have placed limitations on
what we can provide. Help me
have compassion and wisdom to
care for my patients as a
reflection of your love.

※

Action *Plan*:

Research possible grants and prepare a presentation for administration that will benefit your patients.

Prayer 88

PRAYER OVER A LOST PASSION

"For where your treasure is, there your heart will be also."
Matthew 6:21

Lord, I have lost my passion for what I do. Help me discover the zeal I once had so I can revitalize my work for my patients. You promise where I am weak you are strong. I need your strength to carry me today.

Action *Plan*:

Take time to rest. Think about
what excites you now. Has a
shift occurred within you?

Prayer 89

PRAYER WHEN IN NEED OF ANSWERS

"But for you, O Lord, do I wait; it is you, O Lord my God, who will answer."
Psalm 38:15

Lord, we need answers for this precious individual. You know what is wrong and how best to help them. Yet, it seems so elusive. We know there are answers somewhere. Guide and direct us to the answers we need to help this precious person.

Action *Plan*:

Think out of the box to find
creative answers to this
problem.

Prayer 90

PRAYER FOR AN UNHAPPY PERSON

"Judge not, that you be not judged."
Matthew 7:1

Lord, I have done everything I can conceivably think of to make this person happy. Nothing seems to work. I am frustrated and worn out. You know the deep underlying problem in their heart. I give this person to you and ask you to help soften their heart. Show me how to serve them with a smile on my face even when they do not receive the kindness bestowed.

✿

Action *Plan*:

Pray for the person every time
you walk in their room.

RESOURCES

Songs Mentioned:

- "Love Them Like Jesus"
  Casting Crowns
- Leaning on the
  Everlasting Arms
      traditional hymn

Books Mentioned:

Gary Chapman and Paul White
The 5 Languages of Appreciation
in the Workplace
2019 Northfield Publishing

Gary Chapman and Paul White
    Rising Above a Toxic
Workplace: Taking Care of
Yourself in an Unhealthy
Environment
2014 Northfield Publishing

Useful Websites:

Positive Approach to Care
    teepasnow.com

Alzheimer's Association
    alz.org

National Alliance for Mental
Health
      nami.org

*National Suicide Prevention
Lifeline
suicideprventionlifeline.org*

The Five Love Languages
5lovelanguages.com

Diana Leagh Matthews is a writer, speaker, vocalist, Bible teacher, semi-professional genealogist and amateur historian.

She has worked in healthcare for seven years. For over the last five years, she has served as an Activity director at a busy rehab and skilled nursing facility. She is a certified activity director and finishing her certification towards becoming an activity consultant.

Her years in healthcare have given her a heart for others in the field and the stresses and issues faced on a daily basis.

She has also served as a caregiver in numerous capacities and has a heart for caregivers and individuals living with dementia.

Leagh {pronounced as L-e-e-} has been published in numerous anthologies including the award-winning Moments with Billy Graham; Pandemic Moments;

Wit, Whimsy, & Wisdom; and Life Repurposed.

At heart she is a novelist and looks forward to the day she can share her stories with the world.

Leagh blogs on hymn histories at DianaLeaghMatthews.com and plans to start a hymn-devo on social media this summer.

CONNECT WITH DIANA LEAGH MATTHEWS

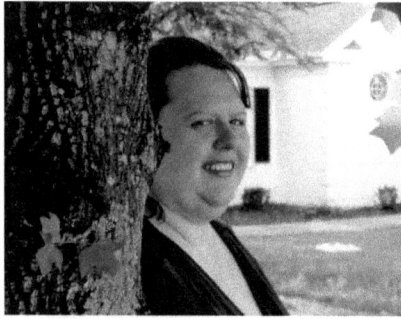

WWW.DIANALEAGHMATTHEWS.COM

DiLeaghMatthews

DianaLeaghMatthews

DiLeaghMatthews

DiLeaghMattthews

DianaLeaghMatthews

Diana Leagh

NOW AVAILABLE FOR
FREE DOWNLOAD

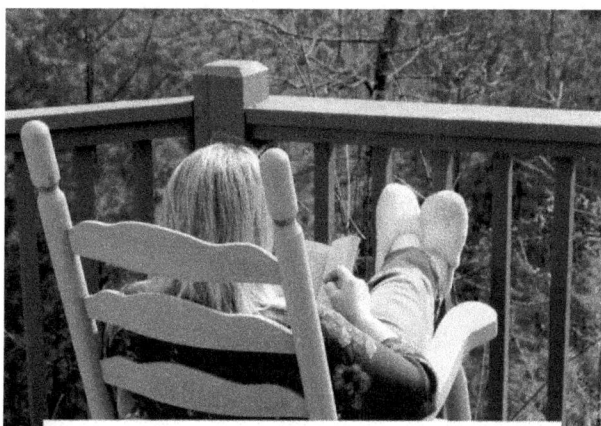

Checklist of
300+ Ways to Find
Renewal

WWW.DIANALEAGHMATTHEWS.COM
/300-WAYS-TO-FIND-RENEWAL/

COMING

SUMMER 2021

Write your own breath prayers

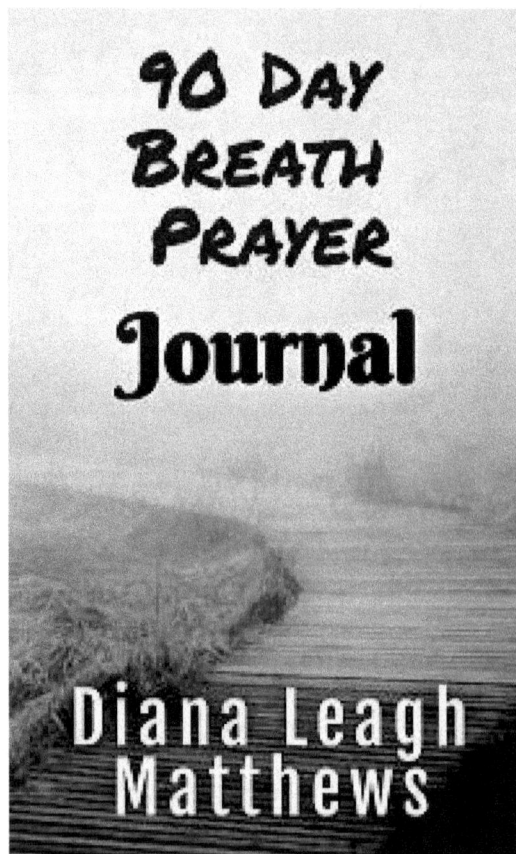

90 DAY
BREATH
PRAYER
Journal

Diana Leagh
Matthews

COMING

AUGUST 2021

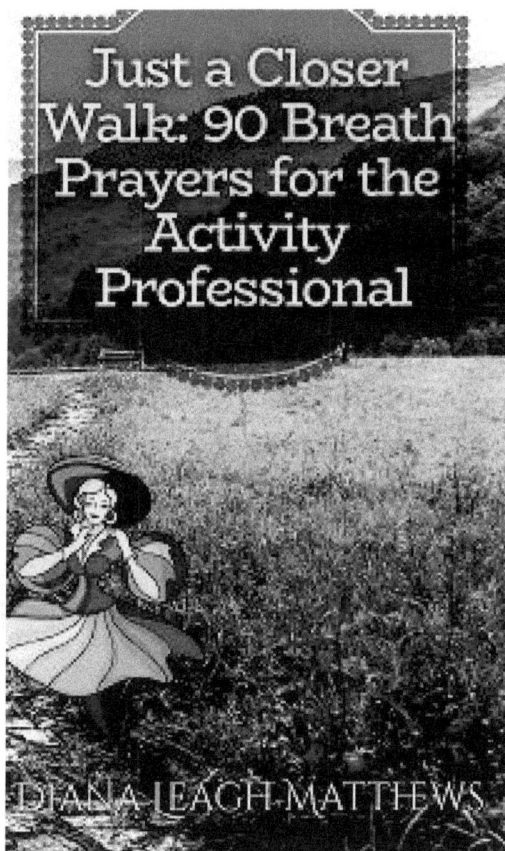

COMING

OCTOBER 2021

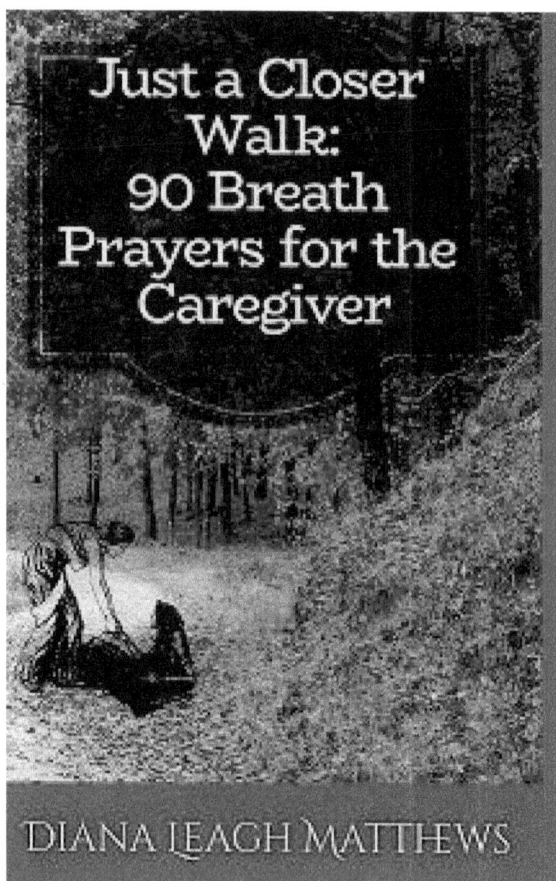

Just a Closer
Walk:
90 Breath
Prayers for the
Caregiver

DIANA LEAGH MATTHEWS

COMING

JANUARY 2022

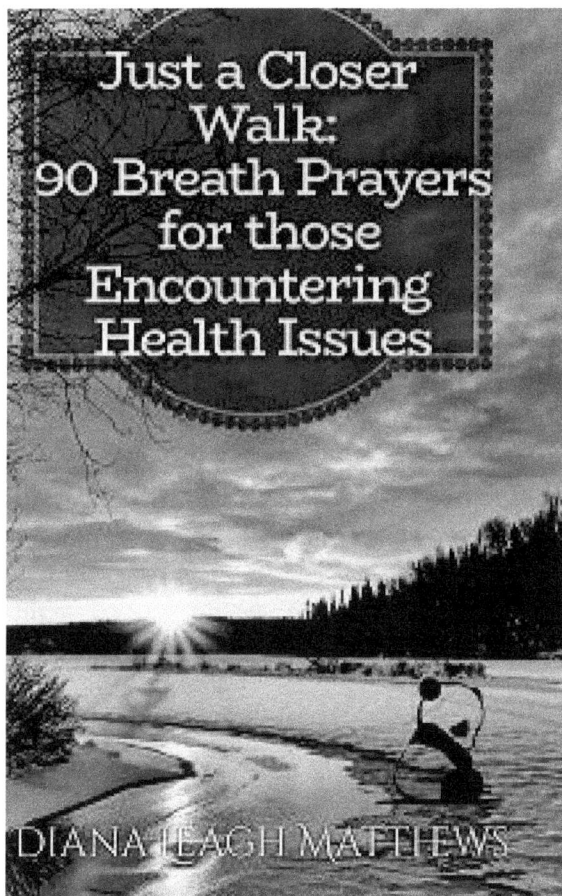

Just a Closer Walk: 90 Breath Prayers for those Encountering Health Issues

DIANA LEAGH MATTHEWS